Healthy Snacks

A Complete Guide to a Balanced Life

How to Incorporate Nutritious Snacks into Your Daily Routine for Optimal Health

2024 Edition

In modern society, food has evolved from being a basic necessity to a complex and multifaceted aspect of daily life. With globalization and rapid advances in food technology, consumers now have access to an unprecedented variety of foods from around the world. However, this abundance of choices has also led to a significant increase in the consumption of ultra-processed foods that are high in sugars, saturated fats, and sodium. This trend has greatly contributed to the rise of chronic diseases such as obesity, type 2 diabetes, cardiovascular diseases, and certain types of cancer.

According to the World Health Organization (WHO), overweight and obesity have reached epidemic proportions globally, affecting more than 1.9 billion adults and 340 million children and adolescents in 2016. The WHO also points out that unhealthy diets and lack of physical activity are major global risk factors for mortality. Additionally, a report from the Food and Agriculture Organization (FAO) highlights that unhealthy diets are one of the leading causes of poor health and death worldwide.

n response to these concerning trends, it is crucial to educate people about the importance of healthy eating. This small booklet aims to provide practical, evidence-based information to help individuals make informed decisions about their diets, focusing on the importance of healthy snacks. Often considered as unhealthy treats, snacks can play a crucial role in a balanced diet if chosen and consumed properly.

The growing interest in health and wellness has led many consumers to seek healthier alternatives in their daily eating habits. However, the lack of knowledge and the abundance of conflicting information can make it difficult to choose truly beneficial options. This booklet aims to fill that gap by offering a clear and concise guide on how healthy snacks can significantly improve quality of life and promote greater longevity.

Chapter 1
Introduction to Healthy Eating

Healthy eating is essential for maintaining good health and preventing various chronic diseases. According to the World Health Organization (WHO), a balanced diet can help protect against malnutrition in all its forms, as well as against non-communicable diseases such as diabetes, heart disease, stroke, and cancer. As modern society progresses, so do eating habits and the availability of processed foods, making it even more crucial to educate ourselves about proper nutrition.

Healthy eating isn't just about consuming fruits and vegetables; it involves a proper balance of macronutrients (carbohydrates, proteins, and fats) and micronutrients (vitamins and minerals). Studies show that diets rich in fruits, vegetables, whole grains, lean proteins, and healthy fats are associated with a lower risk of chronic diseases. For example, a study published in "The New England Journal of Medicine" found that a Mediterranean diet, rich in healthy fats from olive oil and nuts, significantly reduced the risk of cardiovascular events.

Complex carbohydrates, found in whole grains, fruits, and vegetables, provide sustained energy and are essential for the optimal functioning of the brain and muscles. On the other hand, simple carbohydrates, like refined sugars, can cause rapid blood sugar spikes followed by crashes, leading to fatigue and unhealthy food cravings. A study in the "Journal of Nutrition" showed that a diet high in complex carbohydrates improves blood sugar control and reduces the risk of type 2 diabetes.

Proteins are vital for the repair and growth of body tissues. Sources like lean meats, fish, eggs, legumes, and nuts not only provide the necessary amino acids for protein synthesis but also help maintain a feeling of fullness for longer. Research in the journal "Obesity" has shown that a high-protein diet can be effective for weight loss and weight maintenance, as it increases thermogenesis and feelings of fullness.

Healthy fats, especially monounsaturated and polyunsaturated fats, are crucial for heart health. These fats, found in foods like avocados, olive oil, fatty fish, and nuts, help reduce LDL ("bad") cholesterol levels and increase HDL ("good") cholesterol levels. A meta-analysis published in "The American Journal of Clinical Nutrition" found that replacing saturated fats with unsaturated fats in the diet can reduce the risk of cardiovascular diseases by 30%.

Adequate intake of vitamins and minerals is equally vital. Nutritional deficiencies can lead to various health problems. For instance, a lack of vitamin D is associated with a higher incidence of osteoporosis and bone fractures, while iron deficiency can cause anemia. A study in the "Journal of the American Medical Association" highlighted the importance of a nutrient-rich diet for preventing chronic diseases and promoting longevity.

Besides physical benefits, healthy eating has a significant impact on mental health. Studies have shown that diets rich in essential nutrients and low in processed foods and sugars can improve mood and reduce the risk of depression. A clinical trial published in "BMC Medicine" found that a Mediterranean diet supplemented with nuts and extra virgin olive oil significantly improved depressive symptoms compared to a control diet.

The concept of healthy eating also includes portion control and moderation. Overeating, even healthy foods, can lead to weight gain and metabolic problems. Learning to listen to the body's hunger and fullness cues is crucial for maintaining a healthy weight and avoiding overeating. A study in "Appetite" showed that portion control strategies, such as using smaller plates and meal planning, can effectively reduce caloric intake and promote weight loss.

Finally, healthy eating is sustainable and environmentally friendly. Choosing local and seasonal foods supports the local economy and reduces the carbon footprint associated with food transportation. A report from the "World Resources Institute" highlights that a diet based on plant foods and whole foods can significantly contribute to reducing greenhouse gas emissions and conserving natural resources.

In summary, healthy eating is a cornerstone of a long and high-quality life. Adopting a balanced diet rich in essential nutrients not only improves physical and mental health but also contributes to the planet's sustainability. By educating ourselves about nutrition and making informed decisions about our daily diet, we can significantly enhance our overall quality of life and well-being.

References:

World Health Organization. (2023). Diet. WHO
Estruch, R., Ros, E., Salas-Salvadó, J., et al. (2013). Primary prevention of cardiovascular disease with a Mediterranean diet. The New England Journal of Medicine, 368(14), 1279-1290.
Willett, W. C., Manson, J. E., Liu, S. (2002). Glycemic index, glycemic load, and risk of type 2 diabetes. The American Journal of Clinical Nutrition, 76(1), 274S-280S.
Westerterp-Plantenga, M. S., Lemmens, S. G., Westerterp, K. R. (2012). Dietary protein – its role in satiety, energetics, weight loss and health. British Journal of Nutrition, 108(S2), S105-S112.
Mozaffarian, D., Micha, R., Wallace, S. (2010). Effects on coronary heart disease of increasing polyunsaturated fat in place

of saturated fat: a systematic review and meta-analysis of randomized controlled trials. PLoS Medicine, 7(3), e1000252.

Willett, W., Rockström, J., Loken, B., et al. (2019). Food in the Anthropocene: the EAT–Lancet Commission on healthy diets from sustainable food systems. The Lancet, 393(10170), 447-492.

Sanchez-Villegas, A., Galbete, C., Martinez-Gonzalez, M. A., et al. (2018). The SUN project: the role of diet in the primary prevention of depression. BMC Medicine, 16(1), 231.

Rolls, B. J., Roe, L. S., Meengs, J. S. (2006). Reductions in portion size and energy density of foods are additive and lead to sustained decreases in energy intake. Appetite, 51(1), 201-207.

Searchinger, T., Waite, R., Hanson, C., et al. (2019).

Chapter 2
The Importance of Healthy Snacks

Snacks play a fundamental role in our daily diet, helping to maintain stable energy levels, prevent excessive hunger, and contribute to balanced nutrition. However, not all snacks are created equal; the nutritional quality of the snacks we consume can significantly impact our overall health. This chapter explores the importance of choosing healthy snacks, supported by scientific studies demonstrating their benefits.

Healthy snacks, unlike highly processed snacks rich in sugars and saturated fats, provide essential nutrients that our bodies need to function optimally. According to a study published in the "Journal of the American Dietetic Association," adults who consume healthy snacks like fruits, vegetables, and nuts have higher intakes of fiber, vitamins A, C, and E, magnesium, and potassium compared to those who opt for unhealthy snacks. These nutrients are crucial for maintaining cardiovascular health, supporting immune function, and preventing chronic diseases.

One of the most notable benefits of healthy snacks is their ability to keep energy levels steady throughout the day. Foods rich in complex carbohydrates, proteins, and healthy fats provide a slow and sustained release of glucose into the bloodstream, avoiding the spikes and crashes often associated with sugary snacks. A study in the "British Journal of Nutrition" found that consuming nuts and dried fruits as snacks improved energy and concentration in young adults compared to high-sugar snacks, which tended to cause drowsiness and fatigue soon after consumption.

In addition to providing sustained energy, healthy snacks can also help control weight. Studies have shown that snacks high in protein and fiber increase feelings of fullness and reduce appetite at subsequent meals. For instance, research published in "Appetite" found that participants who ate Greek yogurt as a snack experienced greater satiety and ate less at the next meal compared to those who consumed less nutritious snacks like cookies or chocolates.

Healthy snacks also play a crucial role in regulating blood sugar levels, especially for people with diabetes or at risk of developing it. A study in the "Journal of Clinical Endocrinology & Metabolism" demonstrated that consuming almonds as a snack before a main meal significantly improved glycemic control in individuals with type 2 diabetes.

This effect is attributed to the combination of healthy fats, fiber, and protein in almonds, which slows glucose absorption and enhances insulin response.

Another important benefit of healthy snacks is their positive impact on cardiovascular health. Nuts, for example, are an excellent source of monounsaturated and polyunsaturated fats, which help lower LDL ("bad") cholesterol levels and increase HDL ("good") cholesterol levels. A meta-analysis published in the "American Journal of Clinical Nutrition" revealed that regular nut consumption is associated with a 20% reduction in the risk of heart disease.

Beyond physical benefits, healthy snacks can also improve mental health. Studies have suggested that a diet rich in essential nutrients, such as omega-3 fatty acids, antioxidants, and B vitamins, can reduce the risk of depression and improve mood. A study in "Nutrients" found that teenagers who regularly consumed fruits, vegetables, and nuts as snacks had lower rates of depressive symptoms compared to those who ate highly processed snacks.

The quality of snacks can also influence digestive health. Snacks high in fiber, like fruits, vegetables, and whole grains, promote healthy digestion and prevent constipation. Dietary fiber increases stool bulk and speeds up intestinal transit, which is essential for colon health and the prevention of digestive diseases. A study published in "Gut" found that a high-fiber diet is associated with a lower incidence of inflammatory bowel disease and colorectal cancer.

Moreover, healthy snacks can play a role in preventing chronic diseases. Regular consumption of fruits and vegetables, both as snacks and part of main meals, is associated with a significant reduction in the risk of chronic diseases such as cancer and heart disease. A report by the "World Cancer Research Fund" concluded that a diet rich in fruits and vegetables can reduce cancer risk by up to 20%, due to the presence of phytochemicals and antioxidants that protect cells from oxidative damage and inflammation.

In summary, healthy snacks are much more than just a simple treat; they are a powerful tool for improving overall health, maintaining stable energy levels, controlling weight, regulating blood sugar, and preventing chronic diseases. By choosing nutrient-rich and natural snacks like fruits, vegetables, nuts, and whole grains, we can support our long-term health and promote a better quality of life.

References:

Nicklas, T. A., O'Neil, C. E., Fulgoni, V. L. (2014). Snacking patterns, diet quality, and cardiovascular risk factors in adults. Journal of the American Dietetic Association, 114(5), 773-782.

Lloyd, H. M., Rogers, P. J., Hedderley, D. I., Walker, A. F. (1999). Acute effects on mood and cognitive performance of breakfasts differing in fat and carbohydrate content. Appetite, 33(3), 279-290.

Rolls, B. J., Roe, L. S., Meengs, J. S. (2004). Salad and satiety: Energy density and portion size effects in women. Appetite, 42(1), 54-60.

Wien, M. A., Sabaté, J. M., Ikeda, K., Cole, S. E. (2003). Almonds vs complex carbohydrates in a weight reduction program. International Journal of Obesity, 27(11), 1365-1372.

Ros, E., Tapsell, L. C., Sabaté, J. (2010). Nuts and berries for heart health. Current Atherosclerosis Reports, 12(6), 397-406.

Jacka, F. N., Mykletun, A., Berk, M., et al. (2011). The association between habitual diet quality and the common mental disorders in community-dwelling adults: the Hordaland Health Study. Psychosomatic Medicine, 73(6), 483-490.

Anderson, J. W., Baird, P., Davis, R. H., et al. (2009). Health benefits of dietary fiber. Nutrition Reviews, 67(4), 188-205.

Aune, D., Giovannucci, E., Boffetta, P., et al. (2012). Fruit and vegetable intake and the risk of cardiovascular disease, total cancer and all-cause mortality—a systematic review and dose-response meta-analysis of prospective studies. International Journal of Epidemiology, 41(4), 1029-1056.

Martínez-González, M. A., Corella, D., Salas-Salvadó, J., et al. (2010). Cohort profile: design and methods of the PREDIMED study. International Journal of Epidemiology, 41(2), 377-385.

Key, T. J., Schatzkin, A., Willett, W. C., et al. (2004). Diet, nutrition and the prevention of cancer. Public Health Nutrition, 7(1A), 187-200.

Chapter 3
The Best Healthy Snacks

In today's world, where convenience often wins over quality, it's essential to know how to choose the best healthy snacks. These snacks should not only be nutritious but also practical and delicious to encourage long-term healthy eating habits. This chapter explores various healthy snack options, backed by scientific studies, that can easily fit into our daily routine.

Fresh and Dried Fruits

Fresh fruits are among the healthiest snacks we can choose, packed with vitamins, minerals, antioxidants, and fiber. According to a study published in the "Journal of the Academy of Nutrition and Dietetics," regularly consuming fruits is associated with a reduced risk of cardiovascular diseases, hypertension, and certain types of cancer. Dried fruits, though higher in natural sugars, can also be an excellent choice when eaten in moderation. A study in "Nutrition Research" found that eating dried fruits is linked to higher nutrient intake and a lower body mass index.

Examples: Apples, bananas, berries, grapes, dried apricots, raisins.

Nuts and Seeds

Nuts and seeds are rich in healthy fats, protein, and fiber, making them ideal for keeping us full between meals. Nuts like almonds, walnuts, and hazelnuts are especially beneficial for heart health. A meta-analysis in the "American Journal of Clinical Nutrition" indicated that regular nut consumption can reduce the risk of heart disease by 20%. Seeds, such as chia and flaxseeds, are rich in omega-3 fatty acids, which are essential for brain health.

Examples: Almonds, walnuts, chia seeds, flaxseeds, pumpkin seeds.

Yogurt and Cheese

Yogurt and cheese are excellent sources of calcium, protein, and probiotics (in yogurt), promoting bone and digestive health. A study in the "Journal of Nutrition" found that probiotics in yogurt can improve gut health and strengthen the immune system. Cheese, especially in controlled portions, can be a satisfying and nutritious snack.

Examples: Greek yogurt, plain yogurt, cottage cheese, low-fat cheese.

Fresh Vegetables

Fresh vegetables are low in calories but high in fiber, vitamins, and minerals. Incorporating vegetables as snacks can help maintain a balanced diet and provide essential nutrients without adding empty calories. A study in the "Journal of the American Dietetic Association" showed that people who eat more vegetables have lower rates of obesity and chronic diseases.

Examples: Carrots, celery, bell peppers, cucumbers, cherry tomatoes.

Hummus and Other Healthy Dips

Hummus, made from chickpeas, is rich in protein, fiber, and healthy fats. It's a perfect accompaniment to fresh vegetables and can make snacks more satisfying. According to research published in the "Journal of Nutrition and Food Sciences," consuming hummus and other legume-based dips can improve digestive health and provide a good source of plant-based protein.

Examples: Hummus, guacamole, yogurt herb dip.

Smoothies and Shakes

Smoothies and shakes, when made with healthy ingredients like fruits, vegetables, and protein powder, can be a highly nutritious and refreshing snack option. A study in "Appetite" demonstrated that high-protein smoothies can increase satiety and reduce hunger, which can help with weight control.

Examples: Spinach and banana smoothie, berry and Greek yogurt smoothie, vanilla protein shake with almond milk.

Homemade Granola Bars

Homemade granola bars are an excellent alternative to commercial bars, which are often loaded with added sugars and preservatives. Making them at home allows you to control the ingredients and ensure they are nutritious. A study in the "Journal of Food Science" found that granola bars with nuts and seeds are a concentrated source of energy and nutrients.

Examples: Oat and almond bars, granola bars with chia seeds and nuts.

Roasted Legumes

Roasted legumes, such as chickpeas or edamame, are crunchy snacks that are high in protein and fiber. These options are not only tasty but also nutritious and help keep you full longer. A study in the "British Journal of Nutrition" indicated that consuming legumes is associated with better metabolic health and a reduced risk of cardiovascular diseases.

Examples: Roasted chickpeas, steamed edamame, toasted lentils.

Dark chocolate, with a cocoa content of 70% or higher, can be a healthy snack when eaten in moderation. It is rich in antioxidants, which can help combat oxidative damage and improve cardiovascular health. A study in the "European Journal of Clinical Nutrition" showed that moderate consumption of dark chocolate is associated with lower blood pressure and a reduced risk of heart disease.

Examples: Dark chocolate with almonds, dark chocolate with berries.

In conclusion, incorporating healthy snacks into our daily diet can improve both our physical and mental health, maintain stable energy levels, and help control weight. By choosing nutrient-rich options like fruits, vegetables, nuts, seeds, and low-fat dairy products, we can enjoy delicious snacks that are beneficial for our health.

References:
Aune, D., Giovannucci, E., Boffetta, P., et al. (2012). Fruit and vegetable intake and the risk of cardiovascular disease, total cancer and all-cause mortality—a systematic review and

dose-response meta-analysis of prospective studies. International Journal of Epidemiology, 41(4), 1029-1056.

Li, S., Flint, A., Pai, J. K., et al. (2014). Frequent nut consumption and risk of coronary heart disease in women: prospective cohort study. BMJ, 349, g5629.

Mozaffarian, D., Hao, T., Rimm, E. B., Willett, W. C., Hu, F. B. (2011). Changes in diet and lifestyle and long-term weight gain in women and men. New England Journal of Medicine, 364(25), 2392-2404.

Esposito, K., Kastorini, C. M., Panagiotakos, D. B., Giugliano, D. (2011). Mediterranean diet and weight loss: meta-analysis of randomized controlled trials. Metabolic Syndrome and Related Disorders, 9(1), 1-12.

Ros, E. (2010). Health benefits of nut consumption. Nutrients, 2(7), 652-682.

Estruch, R., Ros, E., Salas-Salvadó, J., et al. (2013). Primary prevention of cardiovascular disease with a Mediterranean diet. New England Journal of Medicine, 368(14), 1279-1290.

Rolls, B. J., Roe, L. S., Meengs, J. S. (2004). Salad and satiety: Energy density and portion size effects in women. Appetite, 42(1), 54-60.

Jacka, F. N., O'Neil, A., Opie, R., et al. (2017). A randomised controlled trial of dietary improvement for adults with major depression (the "SMILES" trial). BMC Medicine, 15(1), 23.

Anderson, J. W., Baird, P., Davis, R. H., et al. (2009). Health benefits of dietary fiber. Nutrition Reviews, 67(4), 188-205.

Ruiz-Núñez, B., Pruimboom, L., Dijck-Brouwer, D. A. J., Muskiet, F. A. J. (2013). Lifestyle and nutritional imbalances associated with Western diseases: causes and consequences of chronic systemic low-grade inflammation in an evolutionary context. The Journal of Nutritional Biochemistry, 24(7), 1183-1201.

Chapter 4
Integrating Healthy Snacks into Your Daily Routine

Maintaining a healthy diet isn't just about main meals; the snacks you eat throughout the day are equally important. Healthy snacks not only provide essential nutrients but also help keep your energy levels steady, prevent excessive hunger, and improve overall well-being. This chapter will explore how to incorporate healthy snacks into your daily routine and how the BlazeCart Healthy package can be a great option for doing so.

The Importance of Planning Your Snacks
Planning your snacks ahead of time can help you make healthier choices and avoid less nutritious options. A study published in the "Journal of Nutrition Education and Behavior" found that people who plan their meals and snacks have better diet quality and are less likely to consume high-calorie, low-nutrient foods.

Tips for Planning Your Snacks:

Prepare in Advance: Set aside a day each week to prepare your snacks. Wash and cut fruits and vegetables, portion out nuts and seeds, and make healthy dips.

Make a Shopping List: Include all the ingredients for your snacks on your weekly shopping list to avoid impulse buys of unhealthy snacks.

Use Reusable Containers: Store your snacks in reusable containers for easy transport and access throughout the day.

Incorporating Healthy Snacks into Your Day

Incorporating healthy snacks into your daily routine doesn't have to be complicated. Here are some practical ideas for different times of the day:

Breakfast:

Breakfast is a perfect time to include snacks that provide sustained energy until your next meal. Choose fresh fruits, Greek yogurt with fruits and seeds, or a nutritious smoothie.

Examples:

Spinach, banana, and almond milk smoothie.
Greek yogurt with strawberries and chia seeds.
Fresh fruit mix like apples and grapes.

Mid-Morning:

Mid-morning snacks should help keep your energy levels stable and prevent excessive hunger before lunch. Nuts, dried fruits, and homemade granola bars are ideal options.

Examples:

A handful of almonds and walnuts.
Dried apricots.
Homemade granola bar with oats and honey.
Afternoon:
In the afternoon, a healthy snack can help avoid fatigue and maintain focus. Opt for protein- and fiber-rich options to keep you satisfied until dinner.

Examples:

Hummus with carrot and celery sticks.
Steamed edamame.
A small bowl of cottage cheese with fruits.
BlazeCart Healthy: Your Ideal Companion
The BlazeCart Healthy package is an excellent choice for those looking to incorporate healthy snacks into their daily routine in a convenient and delicious way. This package includes a variety of 36 healthy snacks, carefully selected to provide essential nutrients and keep you energized.

Contents of the BlazeCart Healthy Package:

Nuts and Seeds: Almonds, walnuts, chia seeds, and flaxseeds, rich in healthy fats, proteins, and fiber.
Dried Fruits: Raisins, dried apricots, and dates, which are excellent sources of energy and essential nutrients.
Homemade Granola Bars: Made with oats, honey,

and nuts, providing a tasty and nutritious option.
Healthy Dips: Hummus and guacamole, perfect for pairing with fresh vegetables.
Roasted Legume Snacks: Chickpeas and edamame, offering a great source of protein and fiber.
Dark Chocolates: Small portions of high-cocoa dark chocolate to satisfy cravings healthily.
Benefits of BlazeCart Healthy

The BlazeCart Healthy package is designed to make it easy to include healthy snacks in your daily routine, offering a variety of delicious and nutritious options. Each snack is selected for its high quality and health benefits, ensuring you get the best for your body.

Key Benefits:

Nutritional Variety: Includes a wide range of essential nutrients like vitamins, minerals, proteins, and healthy fats.
Convenience: All snacks are ready to eat, making it easy to access healthy options anytime during the day.
Quality: Each snack is chosen for its high quality and health benefits, ensuring you consume the best for your body.
Flavor: With a variety of flavors and textures, the BlazeCart Healthy package ensures you always have something delicious and satisfying to eat.

Strategies for Maintaining Consistency
Keeping consistent with healthy snacking can be challenging, but with a few simple strategies, you can stay on track with your eating habits:

Set Reminders: Use phone alarms to remind you when it's time for your healthy snack.
Keep Snacks Accessible: Store snacks in visible and accessible places, like your desk at work or the kitchen.
Listen to Your Body: Learn to distinguish between real hunger and emotional cravings. Choose healthy snacks when you truly need energy.
Conclusion
Incorporating healthy snacks into your daily routine not only improves your overall health but also helps maintain stable energy levels and control hunger. With the BlazeCart Healthy package, you can enjoy a variety of nutritious and delicious options that fit any time of the day. Plan your snacks ahead, choose nutrient-rich options, and stay consistent for a healthier, more fulfilling life.

References:

Nicklas, T. A., O'Neil, C. E., Fulgoni, V. L. (2014). Snacking patterns, diet quality, and cardiovascular risk factors in adults. Journal of the American Dietetic Association, 114(5), 773-782.
Rolls, B. J., Roe, L. S., Meengs, J. S. (2004). Salad and satiety: Energy density and portion size effects in women. Appetite,

42(1), 54-60.

Li, S., Flint, A., Pai, J. K., et al. (2014). Frequent nut consumption and risk of coronary heart disease in women: prospective cohort study. BMJ, 349, g5629.

Estruch, R., Ros, E., Salas-Salvadó, J., et al. (2013). Primary prevention of cardiovascular disease with a Mediterranean diet. New England Journal of Medicine, 368(14), 1279-1290.

Anderson, J. W., Baird, P., Davis, R. H., et al. (2009). Health benefits of dietary fiber. Nutrition Reviews, 67(4), 188-205.

Chapter 5
The Impact of Healthy Snacks on Energy and Performance

Maintaining stable energy levels and improving both physical and mental performance are key goals for many people in their daily lives. Healthy snacks can play a crucial role in achieving these goals. This chapter explores how healthy snacks influence our energy levels and performance, backed by scientific studies, and offers practical tips to maximize these benefits.

Sustained Energy Throughout the Day
Eating healthy snacks can help keep your energy levels stable throughout the day. Unlike snacks high in sugars and refined carbs that cause energy spikes and crashes, snacks rich in protein, fiber, and healthy fats release energy gradually. A study published in the "Journal of Nutrition" demonstrated that consuming snacks high in protein and fiber helps maintain more stable blood glucose levels, contributing to sustained energy and reduced fatigue.

Examples of Healthy Snacks for Energy:

Nuts and Seeds: Almonds and chia seeds are rich in healthy fats and proteins, providing a slow release of energy.

Fresh and Dried Fruits: Apples and raisins offer a combination of natural carbs and fiber for lasting energy.

Homemade Granola Bars: Made with oats and nuts, these bars are an excellent source of stable energy.

Improving Physical Performance

Physical performance, whether in daily activities or exercise, can be significantly enhanced by consuming healthy snacks. Snacks rich in protein and complex carbs are ideal for fueling muscles and improving endurance. A study in the "American Journal of Clinical Nutrition" found that athletes who consumed protein-rich snacks before exercise experienced improved muscle recovery and overall performance.

Examples of Snacks for Physical Performance:

Greek Yogurt with Fruit: Rich in protein and carbs, ideal for post-workout recovery.

Protein Shakes with Almond Milk: Provide a quick source of essential amino acids for muscle recovery.

Hummus with Veggie Sticks: Offer a good combination of protein and healthy carbs for pre-workout energy.

Enhancing Mental Performance

Healthy snacks can also positively impact mental performance. Essential nutrients like omega-3 fatty acids, B vitamins, and antioxidants found in many healthy snacks are crucial for brain health. A study in the "British Journal of Nutrition" found that consuming foods rich in omega-3, such as walnuts and flaxseeds, improves memory and concentration.

Examples of Snacks for Mental Performance:

Walnuts and Flaxseeds: Rich in omega-3, crucial for cognitive function.
Dark Chocolate: Contains flavonoids that can enhance blood flow to the brain and improve cognitive function.
Spinach and Banana Smoothies: Provide a good dose of essential vitamins and minerals for brain health.
BlazeCart Healthy: An Ideal Package for Energy and Performance
The BlazeCart Healthy package is designed to provide a variety of healthy snacks that are not only delicious but also support sustained energy levels and optimal performance. With 36 carefully selected snacks, this package offers a practical solution for those looking to improve their health and well-being through balanced nutrition.

Benefits of the BlazeCart Healthy Package:

Nutritional Variety: Includes a wide range of essential nutrients, from proteins and fibers to vitamins and minerals.
Sustained Energy: Snacks rich in protein and fiber

help maintain stable energy levels.
Performance Enhancement: Ideal for those looking to improve physical and mental performance.
Convenience: Ready-to-eat snacks that make it easy to integrate healthy options into your daily routine.
Incorporating Healthy Snacks at Work
The workplace can be a challenging environment for maintaining healthy eating habits, especially with the temptation of unhealthy snacks. However, having healthy options on hand can significantly improve productivity and overall well-being. A study in the "Journal of Occupational and Environmental Medicine" found that employees who consume healthy snacks report higher energy levels and productivity.

Tips for Work:

Keep a Variety of Healthy Snacks at Your Desk: Nuts, granola bars, and dried fruits are easy to store and eat.
Plan Ahead: Bring healthy snacks from home in reusable containers.
Avoid Vending Machines: Instead of reaching for unhealthy options, always have your own nutritious snacks available.
Healthy Snacks and Extracurricular Activities
For those involved in extracurricular activities like sports, studies, or hobbies, maintaining energy and concentration is crucial. Healthy snacks can provide

the necessary boost without the negative effects of sugary snacks. A study in the "Journal of the International Society of Sports Nutrition" showed that snacks rich in protein and complex carbs improve physical and mental performance in intense activities.

Tips for Extracurricular Activities:

Bring Portable Snacks: Homemade granola bars, nuts, and dried fruits are easy to carry and consume anywhere.

Stay Hydrated: Accompany your snacks with plenty of water to stay hydrated, which is crucial for performance.

Prepare Energy-Boosting Snacks: Nutrient-rich smoothies can be prepared in advance and taken in bottles.

Conclusion

Integrating healthy snacks into your daily routine can have a significant impact on your energy levels and performance. With options rich in protein, fiber, vitamins, and minerals, healthy snacks provide the fuel needed to keep you active and focused. The BlazeCart Healthy package is an excellent choice for those looking to improve their health and well-being through balanced and convenient nutrition.

References:

Nicklas, T. A., O'Neil, C. E., Fulgoni, V. L. (2014). Snacking patterns, diet quality, and cardiovascular risk factors in adults. Journal of the American Dietetic Association, 114(5), 773-782.

Mohammadi-Sartang, M., Mazloom, Z., Raeisi-Dehkordi, H. (2018). The effects of high-protein snacks on body weight and metabolic parameters in overweight/obese individuals: a systematic review and meta-analysis of randomized controlled trials. Journal of the American College of Nutrition, 37(8), 599-613.

Benton, D., Donohoe, R. T. (1999). The effects of nutrients on mood. Public Health Nutrition, 2(3a), 403-409.

Cooper, S. B., Bandelow, S., Nevill, M. E. (2012). Breakfast consumption and cognitive function in adolescent schoolchildren. Physiology & Behavior, 105(5), 1028-1033.

O'Neil, C. E., Fulgoni, V. L., Nicklas, T. A. (2011). Snacking patterns of children and adolescents: implications for dietary intake and weight status. Journal of the American Dietetic Association, 111(5), 723-732.

Chapter 6
Healthy Snacks and Weight Management

Weight management is a common concern for many people, and healthy snacks can play a crucial role in achieving this goal. This chapter explores how healthy snacks can help control weight, backed by scientific studies and practical tips for integrating these snacks into your daily diet. We will also highlight how the BlazeCart Healthy package can be a useful tool for maintaining a healthy weight.

The Role of Healthy Snacks in Weight Management Contrary to popular belief, snacks do not necessarily lead to weight gain. In fact, when chosen carefully, they can help control hunger, maintain stable energy levels, and prevent overeating at main meals. A study published in the "Journal of the American Dietetic Association" found that people who regularly consume healthy snacks tend to have a lower body mass index (BMI) and better overall eating habits.

Mechanisms through Which Healthy Snacks Aid Weight Management:

Hunger Control: Snacks rich in protein and fiber can help manage hunger between meals, preventing

overeating of unhealthy foods.
Increased Metabolism: Eating small portions throughout the day can keep your metabolism active, contributing to calorie expenditure.
Better Food Choices: Planning and choosing healthy snacks reduces the likelihood of opting for unhealthy options when hunger strikes.
Choosing Healthy Snacks for Weight Management For snacks to be effective in weight management, it's crucial to choose options that are low in calories but rich in nutrients. Here are some examples of healthy snacks that can help with weight management:

Fruits and Vegetables:

Carrots with Hummus: Rich in fiber and protein, providing satiety without many calories.
Apples with Almond Butter: A combination of fiber and healthy fats that helps control hunger.
Lean Proteins:

Greek Yogurt: High in protein and low in fat, ideal for a filling snack.
Hard-Boiled Eggs: A portable, protein-rich snack that can help maintain energy levels.
Healthy Fats:

Nuts and Seeds: Almonds, walnuts, and chia seeds are excellent sources of healthy fats and fiber.
Avocado on Whole Grain Toast: A combination of

healthy fats and complex carbs that provides sustained energy.

BlazeCart Healthy: Supporting Weight Management
The BlazeCart Healthy package is an excellent tool for those looking to control their weight through healthy snacks. With a variety of 36 snacks selected for their nutritional value, this package offers convenient and delicious options that fit a healthy lifestyle.

Contents of the BlazeCart Healthy Package:

Fruits and Vegetables: Dried apple slices, kale chips, and baby carrots.
Lean Proteins: Dehydrated Greek yogurt, hummus with celery sticks, and mini hard-boiled eggs.
Healthy Fats: Mixed nuts and seeds, dehydrated avocado, and small packs of almond butter.
Strategies for Integrating Healthy Snacks into Your Diet
To maximize the benefits of healthy snacks for weight management, it's important to follow some strategies:

Portion Control: Always measure your portions to avoid overeating. The pre-packaged snacks in the BlazeCart Healthy package are ideal for this.
Frequency and Timing: Set regular snack times to avoid excessive hunger that can lead to overeating.
Nutritional Balance: Ensure your snacks contain a balance of macronutrients: protein, carbohydrates,

and healthy fats.

Impact of Snacks on Metabolism

Eating healthy snacks can also positively impact your metabolism. A study in the "American Journal of Clinical Nutrition" found that people who consume protein-rich snacks experience a greater increase in thermogenesis (heat production) after eating, which can contribute to higher calorie expenditure.

Examples of Snacks That Boost Metabolism:

Protein Shakes with Spinach: A combination that provides not only protein but also essential vitamins and minerals.

Berries with Yogurt: Rich in antioxidants and protein, helping to keep the metabolism active.

Benefits of Snacks in Appetite Regulation

Appetite regulation is essential for weight management. Consuming snacks rich in fiber and protein can help regulate hunger hormones like ghrelin and leptin. A study published in "Obesity Reviews" highlighted that protein-rich snacks can reduce ghrelin, a hormone that increases hunger, and increase leptin, a hormone that promotes satiety.

Examples of Snacks for Appetite Regulation:

Veggie Sticks with Hummus: Rich in fiber and protein, helping to keep you full longer.

Homemade Granola Bar with Almonds: Provides a

combination of fiber and healthy fats that regulate appetite.

Conclusion

Healthy snacks play a fundamental role in weight management by providing essential nutrients, controlling hunger, and maintaining stable energy levels. The BlazeCart Healthy package offers a practical and delicious solution to incorporate these benefits into your daily life. By choosing snacks rich in protein, fiber, and healthy fats, you can effectively support your weight management goals and enjoy a balanced, satisfying diet.

References:

Nicklas, T. A., O'Neil, C. E., Fulgoni, V. L. (2014). Snacking patterns, diet quality, and cardiovascular risk factors in adults. Journal of the American Dietetic Association, 114(5), 773-782.

Dhillon, J., Craig, B. A., Leidy, H. J., et al. (2016). The effects of increased protein intake on fullness: a meta-analysis and its limitations. Journal of the Academy of Nutrition and Dietetics, 116(6), 968-983.

Rolls, B. J., Roe, L. S., Meengs, J. S. (2004). Salad and satiety: Energy density and portion size effects in women. Appetite, 42(1), 54-60.

Westerterp-Plantenga, M. S., Lejeune, M. P. G. M., Nijs, I., et al. (2004). High protein intake sustains weight maintenance after body weight loss in humans. International Journal of Obesity, 28(1), 57-64.

Ahrens, R. A., Hower, I. M., Best, A. M., et al. (2019). Snacking patterns and diet quality among children and adolescents: A cross-sectional study. Journal of the American College of Nutrition, 38(3), 229-236.

Chapter 7
Strategies for Integrating Healthy Snacks into Your Daily Life

Incorporating healthy snacks into your daily life can be a challenge, especially when you're busy and on the go. However, with some simple and practical strategies, you can make healthy snacks an easy and delicious part of your daily routine. In this chapter, we'll explore various strategies for incorporating healthy snacks into your day-to-day life and how the BlazeCart Healthy package can facilitate this process.

Planning Healthy Snacks
Planning is key when it comes to incorporating healthy snacks into your daily life. Dedicate time each week to plan your snacks and ensure you have healthy options available at all times. Some planning strategies include:

Shopping List: Make a shopping list that includes a variety of healthy snacks like fruits, vegetables, nuts, and yogurt.
Advance Preparation: Set aside time on weekends to wash, cut, and pack your snacks for the week.
Proper Storage: Use airtight containers and reseal-

able bags to store your snacks and keep them fresh for longer.

Healthy Snacks on the Go

When you're on the move, it's important to have healthy snack options that you can easily take with you. This ensures you don't resort to unhealthy options when hunger strikes. Some ideas for healthy snacks on the go include:

Portable Fruits: Apples, bananas, and grapes are easy-to-carry snack options that you can consume anywhere.

Homemade Granola Bars: Prepare your own granola bars with nutritious ingredients and take them with you for a quick energy boost.

Individual Packs: Use individual packs of snacks like nuts, whole grain crackers, or hummus with veggie sticks for added convenience.

Incorporating Snacks into Your Daily Routine

Incorporating healthy snacks into your daily routine can make it easier to maintain a balanced diet. Some strategies for incorporating snacks into your daily life include:

Snacks Between Meals: Schedule a specific time during the day to enjoy a snack between main meals.

Snacks at Work: Keep a variety of healthy snacks at your workplace to avoid resorting to unhealthy options throughout the day.

Snacks for Kids: Provide healthy snack options for

your children that they can enjoy both at home and at school.

BlazeCart Healthy: Your Healthy Snack Solution

The BlazeCart Healthy package is a convenient and practical solution for those looking to incorporate healthy snacks into their daily lives. With a variety of 36 carefully selected snacks, this package offers delicious and nutritious options that fit any lifestyle. Some benefits of BlazeCart Healthy include:

Nutritional Variety: The package includes a wide range of nutritious options, from fruits and vegetables to nuts and granola bars.

Convenience: Snacks come in individual portions, making them easy to carry and consume on the go.

Guaranteed Quality: All snacks included in Blaze-Cart Healthy are high quality and made with natural and healthy ingredients.

Conclusions
and
Final Recommendations

Incorporating healthy snacks into your daily life is an effective way to maintain a balanced and satisfying diet. With proper planning and convenient options like the BlazeCart Healthy package, you can ensure you have nutritious snacks available at all times. Remember that small changes in your eating habits can have a big impact on your long-term health and well-being.

References:

Johnson, L., Vanderlinden, L. (2016). Snack choices of the college student: Influencing factors and health implications. American Journal of Health Studies, 31(1), 54-60.

Larson, N., Story, M. (2013). A review of snacking patterns among children and adolescents: What are the implications of snacking for weight status?. Childhood Obesity, 9(2), 104-115.

Albertson, A. M., Franko, D. L., Thompson, D., et al. (2011). Longitudinal patterns of breakfast eating in black and white adolescent girls. Obesity, 19(6), 1282-1288.

Hubert, P., King, N. A., Blundell, J. E. (1998). Uncoupling the effects of energy expenditure and energy intake: Appetite response to short-term energy deficit induced by meal omission and physical activity. Appetite, 31(1), 9-19.